I0766551

My Son has Crohn's Disease

A Journey through Hell and Back

By: A.G. Lewis

To Jared

We are so proud of the man you are growing
up to be

*For I am the LORD your God who takes
hold of your right hand and says to you, Do
not fear, I will help you – Isaiah 41:13*

Introduction

I struggled with whether to write this book or not. Some of the memories are so painful to relive that part of me just wants to forget them. But, if the horror that our family lived through can help someone else it will be worth the pain of reliving it. Even if this book only helps one desperate parent praying that the doctor can save their child. Or someone who has been diagnosed with Crohn's Disease finds comfort then I will consider this book a success.

I am thankful for all of the great

doctors, support from friends and family and

the miracle of modern medicine that saved

our son. And, I grieve for those who have

not been saved. For those who have a

different ending to their story. For all of the

parents who lose their children every day

because of cancer and other terminal

diseases. We have been truly blessed.

This book is not a medical book and I

am not a doctor. Further, I am not a

professional author I am just a person who

wants to help others by sharing this story.   I

am just a regular parent who never thought

this could happen to our family. So please

forgive any imperfections in format and

spelling. For anyone who is reading this

book who doesn't know the basics of

Crohn's Disease – it is an Inflammatory

Bowel Disease. It is also an autoimmune

disorder like so many diseases today. It

seems to be a little less common than some

of the other diseases of the intestines and

bowels. It is chronic and can effect

different parts of the digestive tract. Our

son's issue is in the small intestines and

honestly I'm not sure if all Crohn's is in the

small intestines. Typically, Crohn's Disease

is managed with diet, medicine and surgery.

It can cause death – mainly from the loss of

blood from bleeding and infection. Most of

the medications work by suppressing the

patient's immune system which increases

the danger of dying from an infection.

Crohn's Disease is often diagnosed in the

teenage to young adult years.

The symptoms that our son

experienced and still experiences when he

has a flare up include abdominal pain, back

pain, diarrhea, blood in the stool or dark

stool, anemia, low blood pressure and a cycle which has become normal of eating and running to the bathroom.

I sincerely thank you for taking time to relive this journey with me. I hope it will enrich your life in some small way and bring comfort to anyone who is living the same journey through hell or to those who have survived it. It is a great compliment for you to spend your time reading my book. Thank you and here we go…

Hindsight is 20/20

When you become a parent you don't receive a manual of how to raise your child. When to advocate and when to trust the doctors. And, like many first time parents we fully trusted that our son's doctors knew far more than we knew. And, that doctors in general were supposed to share our same passion for protecting other people's children. What I have learned over the years is that not all doctors share this vision. There are some really horrible doctors and there are some really great ones. If you find a great one – hang on and don't let go.

Our son was born a happy, chubby and healthy little baby with blond hair, blue eyes and little dimples in his cheeks.   We were such proud parents, quickly our whole world revolved around this little person in our home.   We felt so blessed (and still do) that God gave us such a wonderful son. Looking back, there were some signs early in our son's life that might have indicated to a more experienced parent that a potential digestive problem might exist. But, we weren't more experienced parents. We were

newbies and had a long road ahead of

learning.

When our son was about three months

old he developed Colic. Everyone has

heard the stories of parents driving all over

town during all hours of the night to try and

get a baby with Colic to rest. I can assure

you, I understand parents who go to this

length to try and calm their baby. We

didn't really know it was Colic. We went to

the Pediatrician and told him every detail

and he is the one who told us that our baby

had Colic. He prescribed some "drops" to give to our son when the Colic started to basically take the edge off. To this day, that is one of the scariest medications that I have ever dispensed to my son. We gave him the drops and his eyes just shut – scared me to death. I wasn't sure if he was going to wake up or not. The doctor was correct, it stops the symptoms of Colic because it drugs your baby until the pain is over. I'm not saying it is good or bad I am just saying it was scary. I've read in articles since our son was diagnosed with Crohn's that a lot of babies with Colic later develop diseases that involve the digestive tract. But, we had no idea. And, like I said I am not a doctor the two things may be unrelated. But, my purpose for mentioning it is to warn parents who have a baby with Colic. It could be a warning sign for what lies ahead.

I was fortunate enough to be able to breast feed our son for a short period after he was born. When he went to formula, and this is the second thing I can remember that was an indication of an issue ahead, happened. He would drink the formula and then projectile vomit the formula out. And,

I mean it would shoot like four feet from his body. It was in and then it was OUT. If you have every watched a scary movie from the 1980's it is nothing on watching this formula come flying out of the baby that you love and are in charge of taking care of and protecting. Obviously, this is a concern when the formula is your baby's primary source of nutrients. So, off to the Pediatrician (like all new parents) and we were told that he probably just needed a soy based formula.

Soy formula smells like dog food, FYI. But, we did it and he did seem to keep more of it down. It wasn't a perfect solution but he was maintaining his weight and he made it to the point where he could start on baby foods. We followed all of the rules for introducing baby food. We read everything and followed the instruction down to the last detail. After he started on baby food he would get so constipated (early warning sign number three) I had to bend his legs up toward his chest when we played together to try and get his bowels and gas to move. Pediatrician assured us this was all normal.

Eventually his bowels sort of leveled out for

a while.

	When he went to preschool, I would

come in and ask where our son was?   And,

the three year olds in the class would point

to the bathroom in the classroom. You

know the toilet in all preschool classrooms

that is ten inches off of the ground. I don't

mean this happened once, I mean it

happened almost daily (early warning sign

number four). So, he spent a lot of his

preschool years sitting in the bathroom with

a tummy ache or trying to use the bathroom

or with diarrhea. At this point, probably more constipation that diarrhea. So, we did what we could by sending him apple juice to drink and monitoring his bowels. And, of course we discussed it with his Pediatrician and we were told it was totally normal.

Our son is pale just because my husband and I are fairly pale. But, when I look back at his pictures from baby through high school I can see that he was extremely pale. It seemed normal to us, but in class pictures you can see that the color of his skin was unhealthy. I am assuming that he was missing a lot of nutrients through the years because of the way he digested food. Or, more like didn't digest food. Another thing that he experienced was painful joints as early as elementary school. Somewhere I read that painful joints can be linked to Crohn's as well (early sign number five). I didn't know any of this at the time. Our son had so much pain in his ankle and heel in first grade that we took him to the Orthopedic Doctor. The doctor decided it would be a good idea to put a cast on his foot to try and "rest" his heal. We really weren't provided any huge explanation of why this would help. That was a journey in and of itself. He ended up breaking two casts and a cast shoe before we made it through the six weeks. We were on a first name basis with the Orthopedic Technician "Jack" who patiently put the cast back on each time. Through the years our son's joint pain never went away and it is still something he battles today. He pops and crackles, he can't find a shoe that feels comfortable and if he does too much physically it makes him sick. We simply never realized that this was a potential warning sign for Crohn's Disease. We didn't know to question the doctors who treated him.

The routine of eating and running to the bathroom became normal in our house very early. If we went out to eat we didn't plan on doing anything else before we went home. If we were at home, we knew he was going to go straight to the bathroom. Dinner table to the bathroom. It is impossible to digest nutrients when your food moves through your system that fast. It just became normal. We mentioned it to our Pediatrician who said it was fine. He said it was probably a nervous stomach or

constipation. Trust me, it wasn't

constipation by this point. The doctor

assured us that it was definitely nothing to

worry about. And, so we proceeded day

after day, month after month and year after

year with the same routine. Eat – Poop –

Eat – Poop.   And, we accepted that it was

just how our son's system worked and we

tried to make his life as normal as we could

with this endless cycle of running to the

bathroom.

At this time we had no idea this could

be anything more than his normal way to

digest food. After all, everyone is different.

He was generally happy. He played guitar,

he played baseball, and he played flag

football, built robots with his robotics club

and was a Cub Scout. Despite the

inconvenience, pain and the embarrassment

of his bowel issues he was able to move

forward with a regular life and enjoy being a

kid. We just had to plan when he ate and

when he had to be at extracurricular

activities. We were willing to give the extra

effort to make sure that he could enjoy normal activities.

Looking back at this now, we should have pushed harder to find out what was wrong instead of treating the symptoms. We should have taken him to a Pediatric Specialist who could have tested him to see if he had a disease in his digestive tract. Although, honestly I don't know if they would have found it this early. We thought we were doing all that we could do by helping him cope with his bowels as he grew older.   And, this is where I would say – if you think something is not right with your child then it probably isn't. Don't listen to the doctors who say things are fine. Advocate for your child and don't stop until the source of the problem is found. Also, I just want to mention it is normal for us to mention to our friends and co-workers what is going on with our children. But, when every person you talk to has a horror story of how the same symptoms were cancer or something horrible and the child died. We all know people like this, no matter what you tell them "they" know someone who had it worse or died from it. Don't surround yourself with these people.   Just stop telling

them your personal life. Take care of

yourself and surround yourself with positive

people who love you and want to help.

Ignore the people who have nothing but

negative things to say. It isn't helping you

and it isn't helping your child.

Having said that I can think of two

things my son will tell you right now if you

ask him. And, it is making me laugh right

now just thinking about it. These two things

stem from probably I would guess before he

started school. One time he had chocolate

milk and then threw up. Like, projectile vomited everywhere. I think it is likely that he threw up because he ate too much and not because of the chocolate milk. But, from that day forward if someone said chocolate milk... he said "Chocolate milk makes me throw up." Regular milk is fine... but chocolate milk – too far! The other thing he will say is "I can't have Mountain Dew." I think it did give him a stomach ache once (it has given me a stomach ache more than once), but mainly we didn't give him Mountain Dew because of the sugar – because he turned into a crazy maniac child.

But, all of his years growing up he would tell anyone who offered it to him "My parents said, I can't have Mountain Dew." Indicating that perhaps he had an allergy or something. It's funny how kids interpret what we say. He will be turning twenty one soon and he still doesn't drink Mountain Dew or Chocolate Milk. I hope we haven't caused some sort of childhood trauma that is going to require hiring a Psychiatrist later in life!

The First Symptoms before the Diagnosis

So the digestive issues really weren't anything new by the time our son was fifteen. But, what was new is the back pain. He just started having back pain in the middle of his back. I don't mean it was a little bit sore. I mean horribly painful back pain. When his primary doctor saw him she said the normal things Advil, heat, ice and rest. And, even this early I remember saying – there has been no injury? He hasn't done anything to "pull" a muscle or strain his back. Nonetheless, we followed the doctor's orders. And, in addition we tried everything in the world from essential oils to sports creams. And I am not putting down the efforts of the doctor. We had a great doctor, but they are not psychic. That's why they "practice" medicine. They gather all of the information they can and make their best diagnosis to try and help their patients. Our doctor was not blowing things off, but you expect a digestive problem to hurt in the stomach area. The pain in his back indicated a much different problem. For us too, we had no idea the source was actually in his intestines.

One day we were telling our friend who is an orthopedic doctor about our son's back and he said it just isn't normal for a kid to have such severe back pain at his age. Finally, a doctor agreed. He suggested seeing his colleague who specialized in treating back pain for people of all ages. So, I made the appointment and we went. The first visit, the specialist prescribed a high dose NSAID and suggested buying a new mattress. He didn't even do an x-ray. When it wasn't better in a couple of weeks when we went back he did an x-ray and said it all looked good, increased the dose of the strong NSAID and scheduled an MRI. I get

that most of the time the strong NSAID

should significantly help. When it doesn't it

should be a red flag for the doctor.

We went to the hospital and had the

MRI on my sons back and it showed

nothing. So, more NSAIDS and now

physical therapy twice a week was

prescribed. So, we did it – all of it – every

last thing that the doctor suggested. And,

the pain was getting worse and was

interfering with more and more of our son's

daily activities. His energy level was

horrible and he was in constant pain. He looked pale and he didn't feel good. He was weak and had no stamina. He was having dark stools but I didn't know that at the time. Moms' don't go in the bathroom with their fifteen year old sons. And he didn't know what it meant, he just knew he hurt. Another thing I learned after that fact, is that if you think your child is anemic check their fingernails. If they are white instead of pink, not good. Also, the gums. I didn't have this information at the time and in case it can help anyone else I wanted to mention it here.

I can remember, during this whole

fiasco we were mowing grass one evening

and literally our son just fell down on the

concrete and stayed there. I ran over and he

could barely move, he was dizzy and his

heart was beating superfast. I got him some

water and we got him cooled down and I

knew this was something a lot more serious

than what the back doctor said. Our son

isn't a complainer, and for him to react this

dramatically to the pain in his back. I knew

something very serious was wrong. I didn't

know where he needed to go to get help.

That is a very helpless feeling. Especially

when you have already gone to the doctor and specialists and no one seems to be able to figure out what is wrong. It is actually just terrifying. This was now interfering with his ability to enjoy daily activities. He felt horrible, he was in constant pain and he had zero energy to do daily tasks. This was definitely NOT normal. It was all he could do just to get through the school day. To his credit, he made himself go to school even when he felt horrible.

The eating and running to the bathroom continued. Sometimes he would be in the bathroom for half an hour either trying to use the bathroom or with diarrhea. Almost always after he ate. Fifteen year olds are supposed to eat nachos, pizza and brownies and play video games, mow grass, play with their friends. They are not supposed to be in constant misery. We had to find someone who could figure out what was wrong. Not only was our son miserable, but as a parent it is a horrible feeling not to know what to do to "fix it" and we didn't know what to do to "fix it." We had followed all of the doctor's orders down to the last detail.   We had tried homeopathic treatments. And, this is when things first started to get scary. What if something else was wrong? What if he has cancer? What if he has a spinal problem? Every possible thought crossed our minds. And, meanwhile we are trying to keep a normal schedule with him going to school and us going to work. School absolutely wiped him out. By the time he got home he had nothing left. He had to sleep before he could do homework. He was in all advanced courses and regularly had two to three hours of homework every night.

I can remember one evening he felt horrible so he said he was going to take a shower. He had already been in the bathroom for a long, long time. Looking back, I am assuming he lost some blood when he went to the bathroom.   So he took this long hot shower and when he got out he just fell to the ground and was dizzy. When we took his blood pressure it was very low. After he got cooled down and something to drink, his back was still killing him but his blood pressure became more normal. I think I may have slept in his room that night. I just had a feeling that something horrible was wrong. So, I made another appointment with his primary doctor to try and figure out who he needed to see next. The NSAIDS, physical therapy and rest were not working. In fact, things were getting worse in a hurry and the NSAIDS were not getting rid of the pain. In fact, they weren't really making it that much better. Now, his stomach hurt all of the time, presumably from taking all of the NSAIDS. And, his back was still killing him. He needed help and we needed our doctor to help us find someone who could help.

One thing we later found out from someone at the hospital is that people who have Crohn's Disease should not take NSAIDS.   By NSAIDS I mean aspirin, ibuprofen (Advil) and naproxen (Aleve) and a lot of cold and allergy medications.   Our doctor told us later that NSAIDS can cause flare ups in people with Crohn's Disease and they can make symptoms worse over all. The large dosage of NSAIDS that our son was prescribed were both making the symptoms worse and creating other issues in his body that we didn't know about until later.

911

This is where the part of the book where the horror starts and the part that is hard to relive in these pages. In early December of 2014 our son stayed home from school because he wasn't feeling well. The same stuff he had been dealing with weakness, low blood pressure, and severe back pain and generally feeling horrible. Normally, I would not have stayed home with him at this age, but this illness had been going on for months and months and something told me that I needed to stay home with him. It is that decision that probably saved his life, and is a lesson to all of us that when you have that feeling inside that you should do something – do it.

I wasn't sure that morning if he had some sort of stomach virus or if it was more of the same thing we had been dealing with but I knew he was sick really sick. Mid-morning he said he was going to take a shower. He was in the shower a long time. To the point that I was knocking on the door and asking if he was doing ok? When he got out he just fell to the ground and he was super weak. We got him to his room and he said "I need to go to the hospital." I brought him a Gatorade and we got him cooled down. And, he said I think I need to go to the bathroom. While he was laying on the floor in his room one of the most horrific things I have ever experienced happened.

He threw up a mixture of Gatorade, blood and a huge, huge blood clot. I didn't know what the blood clot was – this will sound stupid but it looked like an organ it was so big. I have no idea how someone can throw up something like that and not choke to death. I tried to take his blood

pressure and could get nothing. I called 911.

        Before I proceed any further I would

like to say that all of the emergency

responders from the person who took the

911 call to the paramedics and fireman who

came to our home were amazing.   Within

two minutes help had arrived at our home.

        So my son was on the carpet in his

bedroom. He was essentially unconscious,

he had a blood clot the size of a stomach

next to him, blood all over the carpet and I

could not get a blood pressure. I knew his

heart was beating but he was in desperate need of medical attention. That's how fast it happened. He was taking a shower and then he was basically unconscious in his bedroom floor.

The fire truck arrived first and they came right in and started checking his pulse. I told the fireman he threw up something terrible and showed it to him. I told him I had no idea what it was and it looked like an organ of some sort and I was scared. And, he looked at me and said – that is a blood clot. A really big blood clot. EMSA arrived within a couple of minutes. At some

point in the midst of the chaos I must have

called my husband and he was home now.

He worked retail and obviously December

isn't the greatest time for him to just pick up

and leave work. But, he could hear the

panic in my voice.

Here is the image that will never leave

my head about the 911 call. I have an

image in my head of our son laying in the

floor of his room with blood around him on

the carpet and SIX people working on him.

He had two IV's and fluid going in before

he could even object to the needles. The

EMSA paramedics and the fireman worked

together like they had been working in an

operating room together for years. It was

incredible to watch and horrifying to watch

at the same time.

I will never forget one of the fireman

had the same name as my son. And, he said

how do you spell Jared and my son was

talking to him. That fireman kept our son

calm with the simplest of conversations and

is nothing short of a hero in my book. That

fireman's name is Jared Crowder and I will

never forget that... never. He was so

incredible to our son. It is easy to forget

that that fireman are heroes every day.

And, this is just one example. And, I will

never forget while they lifted our son onto a

gurney to take him into the ambulance –

Jared Crowder looked at our son and said

"buddy, you need blood."

I really don't think EMSA wanted me

in the ambulance on the way to the hospital.

But, trust me when I say NOTHING was

keeping me out of that ambulance. I

answered medical questions and provided

insurance information on the ride to the

hospital and watched our son just lying there

pale, lifeless and weak.

We live fairly close to the hospital so

the ride didn't take too long. And, there is a

whole process for moving ambulances in

and out of the area at the hospital. There

was some discussion because of his age if he

needed to go to the Children's hospital or

the regular hospital. It was determined that

he would go to the Children's hospital.

If you haven't every ridden in an

ambulance, there is a chaotic sort of walkie

talkie noise. New calls coming in for EMSA drivers, communication with the hospital and it is super bumpy. The person who is driving is trying to get to the hospital as fast as they can through traffic and drivers who don't want to be bothered by a passing ambulance. The person in the back is trying to get everything in order so that the transition into the hospital is smooth. It is a well-oiled machine. I don't think most people think about what a special person it takes to actually work on an ambulance. I can't even imagine what they must see on a daily basis.

While I felt relieved that we were on the way to the hospital and we had paramedics who knew what to do to help our son – I also felt terrified to find out what was wrong. I was horrified by the thought that he might not make it. He may not survive. How can you throw up a blood clot that looks like that and survive? Was that in his stomach? Is that what has been hurting? I had a million questions.

It is amazing how at that moment not one other thing mattered in the world. Not my husband's work that he had to just leave.

Not my new job that I started a few months

earlier. Not our son's schoolwork. Not the

fifteen errands I needed to take care of that

day. Not the dishes in the sink or the

laundry. Not the blood all over my son's

carpet in his room. Nothing. The only

thing that mattered was finding the right

doctor who could save our son. I remember

thinking, please God, save our son and give

the doctors the skill that they need to save

him. Please God, please.

We were probably in the ambulance

less than fifteen minutes but the vivid

memory I have of all that was going on will

never fade away.   Our son was literally

almost unconscious the whole ride.   His

body could not take anymore and it was

trying to shut down.   No fifteen year old

should have to experience something like

this, ever.   We had failed at all of our

efforts to make him well and now we needed

a miracle.

The Emergency Room

When we arrived at the Emergency

Room my husband was already there and he

looked equally terrified by what was

happening. We were immediately taken

back to an examination room.   Our son was

lifted from the gurney to a rolling hospital

bed. The room was white and sterile. There

were monitors for everything you can think

of and our son was hooked up to all of them.

His blood pressure was very low. The dr.

came in right away and our son was started

on several IV medications. They took a

blood sample and we waited.

I can remember, while we waited for

the results of the blood test our son saying. I

can't stay here tonight I have a Calc test

tomorrow. I reassured him that his teacher

would let him make-up the Calc test. At

that point, he didn't realize how sick he

really was or how anemic his body had

become. We didn't either.

The blood results came back and

confirmed that he was extremely anemic.

His hemoglobin was 4.5. At the time I

didn't know how alarming that number was – but I quickly got an education on what a proper hemoglobin number should be. I can remember our primary care physician calling my cell phone and asking what his hemoglobin was and when I told her she wanted me to confirm with the nurse. When I confirmed it she educated me on what it should be and said he needed to be right where he was because he was having an emergency. That part we had already figured out.

While we waited for the doctor to come back in we sat and looked at our fifteen year old son laying on the hospital bed – pale and lifeless. When the doctor came in he said they needed to start a blood transfusion as soon as possible. Since, our son was a minor it required several signatures to get the blood transfusion process started. It's amazing how under normal circumstances you might be worried about the dangers of a blood transfusion. But, in this instance we could not get the blood flowing into his body fast enough.

It is pretty interesting the process of giving a blood transfusion. It goes into the IV as you would expect but the nurse stands there and watches for any side effects or adverse reactions. They time it – like two minutes, five minutes, and ten minutes. And, as soon as that bag was empty it was replaced with another. He had two bags of whole blood before we ever got a room. And, every bag of blood he received gave him itchy eyebrows. It must be normal to get some little weird reaction from someone else's blood because the doctor just ordered Benadryl to help with it. I had no idea.

Some of the bags of blood caused more of a reaction than others.   And, it seems so strange that only his eyebrows were ever itchy. We were lucky, there were no other serious side effects from the blood transfusions.

To put this into perspective our son's hemoglobin was 4.5. A normal teenage boy should have a hemoglobin of about 11-14. And as I understand it anything less than 8 is considered to be anemic.   He was dangerously low on blood and dangerously anemic.

After we had gone through his medications and the treatment he had been receiving for his back pain the doctor determined that he needed to have his stomach pumped. Two reasons – to get all of the NSAIDS out of his stomach and to get the blood out of his stomach.

When our son was a baby I can remember him getting a chest x-ray. Where they put your infant in a clear acrylic form with their hands up and take the x-ray. Meanwhile the baby cries and turns blue. At the time, I thought that was the most horrific thing I would ever see my son go through. I can remember sobbing during and after. And, the treatment that he received afterwards for RSV on his first birthday seemed like the worst thing parents could ever see their child endure. I was wrong.

The process to "pump" someone's stomach starts with, in our son's case, calming the patient down. Although, he was so weak it wasn't much of a protest. And, he was scared and was willing to do whatever he had to do to survive. Next they insert a lubricated tube down the throat,

down the esophagus and into the stomach so

that suction can be applied and the stomach

can be emptied.   Sounds simple enough.

So they start to put the tube down our son's

throat and the gagging and hurling start.

They have obviously dealt with this before

so they tell him to sip some water and it will

help the tube go down. It did, but then the

tube is in your throat and it feels like you are

gagging, gagging, gagging.   Awful. Truly

awful for him and truly awful to watch. We

didn't know at the time that the tube would

be staying for quite a while longer.

I have two positive things to say about that Emergency Room visit. First, it saved our son's life. The knowledge and training that the staff had and their quick action was the difference between life and death for our son. Second, the compassion that the staff showed to us was amazing. They never walked out of the room without asking if my husband and I needed anything. Something to drink or a snack. It was obvious that they cared about what was going on and for our family.

I can't really explain the mix of emotions that were going on in the Emergency Room. And, it was then that I realized we had no idea what was wrong with our son. Our son was scared to death and had no idea why this was happening or what was wrong with him. And, because of that he almost died. He literally almost bled to death while we were following doctors' orders and taking him to physical therapy and feeding him NSAIDS. The doctors were fighting to save his life and we were praying that God would save him.

The Hospital Stay

After you get blood it doesn't immediately make your hemoglobin level rise. So, you get the blood and wait. The nurse takes the blood sample and you wait – then the doctor decides if you need more blood.   At this point we still had no idea what was actually wrong with our son. We knew he threw up a huge blood clot and we knew he was anemic. The doctor had indicated that he thought the issue was a gastrointestinal issue. But, there wasn't a real way to know what was wrong without being able to scope him.

The tube remained and my husband and I watched as the bloody, yellow stomach acid was pumped out of our son's stomach and into a holding container next to his bed. This went on for days. Since his hemoglobin was so low and it wasn't increasing very quickly (indicating he was still losing blood) the doctor couldn't do any type of scope. I believe they needed his hemoglobin to be 9 before they would give him anesthesia and proceed with a scope.

So we waited, his stomach continued to

pump and he was given antibiotics, fluids

and blood through his IV. This went on for

about three days.

     While this process was occurring our

son could not drink, eat or get up. He was

allowed to have Carmex for his dry lips and

Chloraseptic for the gagging feeling from

the tube and for his sore throat from the

tube. We sat in the hospital room. We

tried to watch TV. He was sleeping a lot.

He couldn't get up to go to the bathroom so

he had to use a urinal. When my husband was there he helped him.

I will never forget the first time I was the one there with him when he needed to use the bathroom. And, he was not going to have his mother helping him pee. I reminded him that I had already seen it all when he was a baby. He finally settled for me helping him and after that it wasn't an issue. How humiliating for him to not be able to get up and use the bathroom. The whole thing was like a horrible nightmare that wouldn't stop.

My husband had to be gone from the hospital during the day because as I mentioned earlier he was in retail and it was December. In retail, you get one month to basically make your profit for the whole year. He was checking in and called and stuff but he couldn't just sit at the hospital. He came in the evening and then he went home to take care of our dog.   I had been at my job only a few months. Luckily, I had an amazing boss and I was able to do work from my laptop while I was sitting at the hospital.

I can remember after each blood transfusion our son would get itchy eyebrows. They would give him Benadryl. He would be tired but restless. Since he was in a children's hospital all of the rooms had Johnson and Johnson baby lotion. So I would take the lotion and rub it on his feet and calves to help him relax and go to sleep. When the nurses saw it the first time I don't know if they thought I had finally lost it, if it was sweet or if it was totally ridiculous. They didn't say much. The whole time the pumping kept on and more and more and more stuff came out. We needed the liquid coming from his stomach to be clear so that

the tube could come out and he could be

scoped and checked out. We needed to find

out what was wrong with our baby.

And, the cycle went on – blood, blood

sample, and results. About day four the tube

was able to be removed. He could have ice

chips finally and his hemoglobin was barely

high enough so that he could have his

stomach scoped. Looking back, I have no

idea why the gastrointestinal doctor did not

also scope his colon. I was too traumatized

to question it and I just wanted to find out

what was wrong. I later determined that the Gastro doctor wasn't very good, more on that later.

The results from the scope showed that our son had huge ulcers from the large doses of NSAIDS that the back doctor had been prescribing. And, the blood clot he threw up was actually covering a huge open sore in his stomach. Still no explanation for the back pain. The doctor just sort of chalked it up to – if you had an ulcer that size your back would hurt too.

So, the blood transfusions continued, antibiotics and fluids. I don't think it was until around day 6 that he got to have any type of a liquid diet.   And, he was essentially pain free. No back pain.

After a week in the hospital, it was a weird mix of emotions for me. Yes, I would like to sleep at home. Yes, I need to get back to work. Yes, I am terrified to take him home in case another episode happens. We were eventually released I believe around day 8.

We had a follow up appointment at the "clinic" with the doctor who had scoped his stomach. And, we had two antibiotics, Protonix for his stomach acid and it seems like some sort of liquid medicine that was the equivalent of really strong Pepto Bismal. And, he was supposed to be on a soft food diet. This includes things like eggs, pasta, soup, liquids, and baked potatoes. One thing, our son is a super picky eater. He doesn't eat eggs, no pasta, and no soup. So we were looking at soft rolls and baked potatoes. He did eventually drink chicken broth because he was starving to death but he put about three tablespoons of salt in it to

get it down.

And, so he was released with strict

instructions. He had already missed almost

two weeks of school. He wasn't strong

enough to go to school. He was having a fit

about getting to school because he was

worried about his GPA. So I picked up his

homework so he could try to work on it at

home. The doctors thought he should

probably stay home at least one more week.

Finally Home

While he was in the hospital I had corresponded with several of our son's teachers. They had in turn relayed to the students in his classes how sick he was and my son's favorite teacher came to visit him at our home after he was released. That really meant a lot to our family.   There are not a lot of teachers who go that extra effort and who care for their students in that way. Our son ended up having that teacher all four years of high school for all of his advanced Math courses.

We went to our follow up appointment at the "clinic" with the Gastro doctor who treated our son in the hospital. First, it was a true clinic. It was in a bad part of town. We have insurance, we don't normally go to clinics, and we generally utilize doctor's offices with appointments. But, this was the guy with the results from the hospital and we went. And, we waited and we waited and we waited. Then we were told that an x-ray had to be done before he could see the doctor. So we sat and we waited – wild and crazy kids were running around everywhere with trashy parents who were cussing at them. It was a germ fest.

We got the x-ray and then waited and waited and waited some more. Finally, we were called back to the examination room. The doctor had a picture of an x-ray up and promptly started explaining about what the x-ray showed. Finally, I stopped him mid-sentence and said. Is this the right x-ray? And, IT WASN'T.   And, he wasn't even embarrassed. He just said, oh let me get the right x-ray.   At any rate, his diagnosis was that our son was constipated and that he didn't need to see him again. REALLY? I

missed half a day of work, made my weak

son get out to go to this trashy clinic and

now this was the conclusion.

What if we didn't have insurance?

What if this is the type of medical care you

were forced to endure? I was upset, our son

was upset and obviously we never went

back.

Over the next ten days or so our son

started to get some strength back. And, we

decided we would let him try to go to school

at least part of the days. We had already

received a threatening letter from the school

that he had missed too many days and that

he may be held back because of that –

really? That's just the kind of stress a parent

needs. We have a 4.0 student going through

a crisis and we are receiving threatening

letters from the school.   It was really

insensitive.

He made a couple of half days and he

was slowing getting a little bit stronger.

And, he decided he would go to a study

session at school on a Saturday for Calculus.

Session started around 8:00 am and he did

fine.   They were all having pizza – so he drove home and ate a couple of soft rolls and went back.   That is about the extent of what he could eat at that time.   He had gotten so skinny that he was wearing jeans from when he was in sixth grade.   Don't ask me why they were still in the house.   But, they were and it worked out because all of his clothes were huge on him from not eating.

So he went back for the afternoon session.   As soon as I knew he was safely back at school. I decided I would go get some Christmas shopping done. Christmas was in a few days and I had done zero Christmas shopping between being at the hospital and dealing with work and the house, etc. So I headed to Best Buy. I had a cart full of potential gifts when my phone rang. It was a number I didn't recognize and I almost didn't answer.

When I answered it was our son's Calculus teacher. And, he said "Jared is fine – but he threw up blood and passed out. We have called an ambulance," to which I responded I am on my way. I ran out of

Best Buy, got in my car and drove like

Mario Andretti until I got to the school.

When I parked two kids were in the

parking lot waiting to help me find Jared as

fast as possible. He had blood all over his

face, there was blood all over the carpet in

the classroom. The ambulance paramedic

was gathering information. Our son was

providing his whole medical history and

medication list right in front of his whole

class. The students looked horrified, our

son looked horrified. Like, why? We

followed all of the instructions... why is this happening.

I hopped in the ambulance with him. Left his car and my car in the parking lot. I really didn't care how or if they got home. We went back to the emergency room. I can remember this time the driver trying to take us to the adult emergency room. I kept saying we need to go to the Children's ER. He was treated less than two weeks ago in Level 3 of the Children's hospital. Eventually, the hospital made him take us to the Children's section.

This time, they put us in a room for a potential suicide patient. I still don't know if that's because he came back in so quickly after he was released or if that is all that was available. At any rate, I finally called my husband and he headed to the hospital. He was right smack dab in the middle of his busiest season of the year. And, they did blood work. He was anemic again and was still losing blood. He was admitted to the hospital and his blood level was brought back to normal and he was released after a few days.

We took him to his primary care

doctor who did blood work. And, she

discovered that his Ferritin was extremely

low and suggested finding a better Gastro

doctor.   And, she provided us with a referral

for one. This doctor was a Gastro doctor for

adults but he agreed to take Jared as a

patient.

He questioned why the doctor in the

hospital didn't do a colon scope? I told him

we had no idea. So he did a colon scope

which showed nothing. He said then, he

thought it was Crohn's. But he wanted

another test. So, he sent us to the hospital to

take a test that would show the small

intestines.

Basically, the patient swallows a

capsule that has a blinking light. It is about

the size of a large antibiotic. You wear a

purse type thing all day, eight hours I think.

Then you return the bag. And, well you get

to keep the capsule when it comes out. The

doctor watches the film and looks for any

abnormalities. The doctor said he expected

it to show nothing, but in fact it showed the

source of the back pain. The bleeding was

coming from his small intestines. Finally,

we knew what the source of the back pain

that we originally started treating so long

ago.

Treatment

The basic goal of treatment is to put the disease in remission. Crohn's Disease is an autoimmune disease so basically you need to get the body to stop attacking itself. Generally, this is accomplished through diet, medication and surgery.   I am thankful we did not need the last option.

The disease isn't going away, it is chronic. The first part of our son's treatment was a liquid and soft food diet (minus the rolls that caused the second trip to the emergency room).   He is such a picky eater that his diet really consisted of

apple juice, milk, water, baked potatoes and

Campbell's chicken noodle soup chicken

broth.

It takes about an hour and a half to

bake a potato in the oven. By now, I was

back at work and so was my husband. So I

figured out that a restaurant near us called

Charleston's had curb side pick-up and very

delicious baked potatoes. So that's what I

got lunch and dinner. And, that is what

sustained our son for eight weeks. The

employee at Charleston's finally asked why

I was coming so much about two weeks into the whole event and I told her.   The next time I had Jared with me and she looked at him and said "so, you are the one eating all of these baked potatoes!" He thought it was funny.

When our son returned to school he discovered something very interesting in his Calculus classroom where the study session had been prior to his last visit to the hospital. The stain in front of his chair where he threw up blood was still there. I feel like that could be some violation of health and safety rules, but nonetheless it made our son "famous" at school. And, his teacher let him move up one seat so he didn't have to look at it. Which was very much appreciated. All of the students and teachers were suddenly checking on our son all day. Doing ok? Feeling ok? It was an annoyance to our son, but very much appreciated by his parents.

Lunchtime was tricky – Jared was old enough that he really didn't want me bringing him a milkshake or Charleston's to school while the other kids were eating school lunch. He would get so mad if I just

brought stuff. The issue was, he couldn't go

all day without eating because it made him

sick. He couldn't eat anything at school.

And, he didn't want his Mom bringing

anything.

One of his teachers told me, I don't

care if he eats a milkshake in my class every

single day if it keeps him well. So, this is

one instance where we weren't fighting the

school. Everyone knew he was sick and

they were for the most part being helpful.

He still continued to be weak, pale and

going to school took everything he had – the back pain was better but not gone.

I changed my route to work to include a quick drive by the school in the morning. It isn't very far from our house and I liked to see our son's truck there to be sure he made it safely to school. One morning I drove by and there was an ambulance in front of the school with its lights on and kids all around. I didn't stop but I immediately called the school office crying and freaking out. They said they couldn't tell me who the ambulance was for because of privacy rules.

So I finally said – can you just tell me if it is

for our son? And, probably against several

rules she told me it was for a teacher who

was diabetic.

It is amazing how this whole incident

made our son more dependent on us and us a

lot more protective of him. Suddenly, we all

needed to know where everybody was every

second. The smallest sign and everyone

freaked out thinking the worst was about to

happen.

When we left the hospital after the

second stay in the hospital the Pediatrician

who had been treating him gave me the direct number to Level 3 at the hospital and said to call next time and they would get our son right in – so that we could avoid the emergency room. He said, we already know what is wrong just bring him on up. He had great care at the hospital and overall great doctors. Besides the horrible Gastro doctor, the only other complaint I had was the never ending interns. I know they have to learn, but when you have a patient as sick as our son was at that time – you don't need to be examined 20 times before you see the actual physician. And, they all had a different take on what was wrong. It became such a frustration that I requested no more interns. It was just too exhausting for everyone.

And, so our son survived the eight week diet and slowly was able to eat more. By now, the medicine was really helping and we could see progress. While Jared was on his special diet my husband and I had quit cooking anything at home and eating dinner at home. We would get something on the way or eat something that didn't smell good.   As our son began to heal we were able to eat meals together again.

Infusions

I really didn't know very much about Infusions prior to our son being diagnosed with Crohn's Disease. I guess I knew about them for cancer patients and terminally ill patients but I didn't realize how many patients who have gastrointestinal issues have to get infusions. Really for a lot of different reasons medicine, blood, nutrients.

I learned something while our son was taking these infusions. Your body needs certain things to make new blood. The body needs B12, Vitamin C, Iron and Vitamin A.

Our son still had very low iron and ferritin.

If you take an iron supplement a lot of the

pill is waste and it takes a lot longer to

increase your iron level. Also, iron

supplements often will hurt your stomach.

The NSAIDS that our son had taken while

being treated by the back doctor left huge

ulcers in his stomach. So we weren't only

dealing with the Crohn's – he still had open

sores in his stomach.

If you get the iron through an infusion

it goes directly into your bloodstream and

fills up your level quite fast.   So the doctor

ordered, it seems like three infusions. Let me just explain one thing. It is not simple or enjoyable to convince the insurance company that your sixteen year old needs to be approved for infusions. They had his medical records. They had paid for all of the transfusions. They had the results from the capsule test – yet it took nothing short of a miracle to get the infusions approved. After much debate and persistence they got approved.

Our son has a true phobia of needles. He was not excited about having to get infusion treatments. In fact, I think he was hoping the insurance company would not approve them. So, we arrive at the infusion center. It was very home like. Everyone had a recliner to sit in and TV to watch while they were getting treatment.

We were by far the youngest people in the whole place. The workers were older, the patients were really old. And, here is our son in his school uniform sixteen years old waiting for his infusion.

The nurse would get the needle in and then we would sit and let the iron go in for about an hour. Then he would go to school.

The infusions were probably one of the

things that made the biggest difference in

the amount of time it took our son to

recover. They gave him an energy boost,

his complexion improved and he started

thriving again. He would get the infusion

wait a couple of weeks and then get blood

work. More needles which wasn't very

enjoyable for our son. Then another

infusion and repeat. Finally, his iron level,

ferritin level and hemoglobin level moved

into the normal range. No more infusions.

Those little old lady workers were sad to see him go!

Our son was lucky, a lot of the medications for Ulcerative Colitis and other gastro issues are administered through infusions. Our infusions experience was a short one, but for many it is a life change to repeatedly get infusions.

Medication

After we knew our son had Crohn's

Disease (thank you to our son's amazing

doctor) we had to figure out how to control

it. I say we because it was a group effort our

son, us and the doctor. The doctor was

invested in getting our son's Crohn's under

control. He knew what he had gone

through and he truly wanted to help get

things back to normal. You just don't find

that every day.

First, it is very likely that our son will

be on medication for the rest of his life. He

has cousins on my husband's side of the family who have similar diseases and they will be on medication for the rest of their lives. It just seems like there is an epidemic of autoimmune diseases in the world today.

The basic options are drugs as I understand it (and I am not a doctor so I don't pretend to know everything on this topic) to control inflammation in your digestive area, antibiotics to treat infections, steroids to control swelling and drugs that suppress your immune system.

Our son had moderate to severe Crohn's right from the start so our doctor told us he didn't want to mess around with medications that may or may not work right away. He said the steroids cause a lot of side effects that are undesirable for a teenage boy. He did warn us that after he started a medication that suppresses your immune system there are pages and pages of side effects. You can't take the medication if you get sick. You have to be careful about being around people who are sick (shouldn't be a problem at all in public school) and all of that sounded ok... until this... it is a shot.

The doctor looked right at our son and said – you have to learn how to deal with the shots. It is what will make you well again. The doctor was able to talk our son down off of the ledge in the office. But, the anxiety was extreme while we waited to start the medication. And, he had to be checked for TB before we could start (more blood work).

First, the co-pay was outrageous, obtaining the approval from the insurance company was time consuming and

frustrating and it was an injection. The first
dose required four shots one right after the
next, then two and then the dosages leveled
out to one injection every two weeks. He is
still on this dose. It gives him thirteen days
in between to get brave enough to let me
give him another one.

Getting those first four shots done at
home with a Mom who knew nothing about
giving shots and a son who breaks out in a
sweat at the sight or thought of a needle was
rough. There just isn't another word for it.
My husband had to just hide in the bedroom,

it was so dramatic.   But, IT WORKED.   It

started working right away and our son

started to get his life back.   He learned how

to deal with me giving him the injections

and life continued.

I don't want to pretend there were no

hick-ups. The medication really does have

some really serious side effects. Including

an increased risk for cancer. Also, every

insurance company we have ordered it

through required it to be ordered through a

Specialty Pharmacy. It has to come mail

order and it is refrigerated. So planning

deliveries when you work is tricky. In the summer you have to worry about how warm the medication gets in that Styrofoam cooler they put it in and you have to diligently keep up with the ordering schedule because you can't just run down to Walgreens and pick it up. Well, you could if you wanted to pay $5K a month for it. They don't really advertise that part on the commercial for this drug on TV.

So things were starting to go really great and our son was better. Everyone was starting to recover from the trauma of the blood clot, the blood, the 911 call, the

ambulance and the hospital. Right up to the

point where our son came home with some

sort of upper respiratory infection. I called

and got him an appointment for the next

morning but in the meantime he needed

something to relieve the symptoms. When I

headed to Reasors to get him some medicine

all I could think was he can't have NSAIDS.

If I give him the wrong medicine we are

going right back to where we started.

So, I went to the pharmacy counter and

asked the Pharmacist what cold medicine

was safe for a teenager with Crohn's

Disease. He gave me an idea of what should

not be in the medication I chose and I went

over to the shelf to look.   There was a

young man standing behind the pharmacist

helping ring people up that day.

As I was looking at the labels almost

in tears. The young man from behind the

counter came over to me and said "How

long has your son known he has Crohn's?"

I could tell he had something to say but felt

a little awkward, he couldn't have been

twenty years old. I said we found out in a

dramatic sort of way and gave him the short version of all that had occurred. And, this young man told me he had Crohn's and that he found out in a dramatic way as well. He said everyone he knew that had Crohn's found out in their teenage years and that it was discovered in a very dramatic way. He helped me find the exact medication to get my son through the night until he could see the doctor.

I never knew that young man's name and I never saw him at Reasors again. In fact I haven't noticed a young person like that working in the pharmacy area since that

day. I am certain that young man was an

angel from God to let me know – hey, it will

be ok- other people have survived this and

your family will too.

I will never forget that helpless feeling

standing in Reasors which was very similar

to the helpless feeling at the back doctor

when this whole journey started. Not

knowing what to do, feeling weak,

exhausted and helpless. I know there are

other parents who have felt the exact same

thing. And, that is primarily why I wanted to write this book.

My message is this – keep trying, keep pushing and don't lose hope.   The right doctor is out there, the answers are out there and you ARE strong enough to deal with it. You have to keep advocating for your child until the answers are found. Stay strong.

Stress of Driving

At this point in the journey our son was old enough to drive. He had his license and he had a 1972 truck that he dearly loved. He was feeling really good and was confident it was fine for him to just drive anywhere he wanted. I, on the other hand kept thinking about the blood clot he threw up in his bedroom. And, there was a very real possibility that he could throw up blood and pass out while driving. I could only think about how quickly things went from not bad to horrific.

All of this is beside the point that he

was a very inexperienced driver in a very

old vehicle. So, take the stress of having a

new driver and multiply that times a

hundred. We did agree to some driving and

in exchange I made him agree to wear a

medical alert necklace. So that if he was in

a car accident a paramedic would

immediately know he couldn't have

NSAIDS and that he was on

Immunosuppressant Therapy.

I was so proud of my medical alert

necklace I found. It looked like a dog tag

sort of and you would never, never know what it was unless you really looked at it. Jared was less than thrilled about the whole thing. And, I am positive that he never wore it one time.   Well, $73.00 down the drain.

The days of driving got easier and easier. And, the truck got more and more reliable. And, our son's ability to be independent again really started to improve his self-esteem and his self-confidence. He could finally be a normal teenager.

I mean except for needing to constantly use hand sanitizer, worry about germs and get an injection every other

weekend. A small price to pay for a normal

and healthy life. We pass the hospital our

son spent so many days in every day on our

way home. And, every time we drive past I

thank God we are not spending the night

there and that our son is finally able to live

his life to the fullest.

High School

The reason I wanted to put something

in the book about High School is simply

because I admire our son's ability to

persevere. He missed school only when he

was in the hospital and when he was just too

weak to carry his backpack to go to school.

He didn't try to get out of school like some

kids would. He just knew he had to be

successful at school and he just kept going.

Even with the days he had to miss of

school he kept his 4.0 GPA. And, he

graduated 11th in his class. To me that is

just incredible. And I admire his strength,

his endurance, his positive attitude and his

trust in us to help him get through his

illness.

When our son graduated from High

School a lot of parents were crying and

weeping. I can honestly say, I was happy

beyond belief. First, no more dealing with

the public school system. Second, our son

endured through all of his adversities and

graduated on time. Despite throwing up a

blood clot that looked like an organ, despite

having his stomach pumped for days and

despite almost bleeding to death before we figured out what was wrong.

He is strong. And, he was successful in high school and he will be successful in life.

In our city any student who lives in the area can attend a Community College for two years free. Jared really wasn't ready to move out and we weren't really sure enough about his stability on the medicine for him to move very far away. And, because of the possibility of getting very seriously ill living in the dorms we all decided together that he would stay home at least one year and then

we would re-evaluate. That one year ended

up being two years. But, he had great

instructors and he had a really good

internship while he was living at home.

He had some time to just do things he

loves – like work on his truck and weld

things. Just time to heal from everything

that he had endured the last couple of years

of high school.   He was close to the doctors

so when he got sick we could immediately

get him in without having to drive and get

him first. It was a good transition time for all of us.

He kept healing and started to fill out and look healthy. And, the episodes of running to the bathroom became fewer and fewer. I can remember asking the doctor if it was normal – the weight he was gaining. And, the doctor reminded me that he wasn't absorbing any nutrients from his food before and now he was actually getting nutrients.

I can promise you I will never complain about his weight. I have never been so happy to see someone gain some weight.   Good bye skinny, sickly kid and

hello awesome!

Moving Away

After the two years at Community College it was time to face reality. Our son was ready to move out. He decided on a smaller school in a somewhat rural area called Stillwater, Oklahoma – Oklahoma State University. He was now a cowboy.

It wasn't practical for him to have roommates because of the immune system issue – so he found a very nice brand new studio apartment. I was happy that it had an alarm. He chose the third floor and I think he has lived to regret that decision.

His health is stabilized and he is an independent, healthy (with the medicine) young man. He is everything you could want your son to be including responsible and kind. He does what he is supposed to do and he cares about others.

Selfishly, I am glad he can't stand to do his own injections. It means I get to see him at least every two weeks. And, that makes Mom and Dad happy.

Will I ever stop worrying – probably not. Will I ever forget what we have gone through together – never! But, I am grateful for the blessing we were given and the

success of his treatment.   When he was in

the hospital we didn't know if he was even

going to make it to the next day. And, now

he has his whole life in front of him. We are

so proud of him.

Conclusion

I hope our journey will help someone else who is facing the same battle.   There is hope! You have to believe there is always hope.   You have to keep trying and never give up.   Hang in there another day and find the answers.   Don't stop until you get the help you need.

Ask others for help, but make sure you are not surrounding yourself with negativity. None of this is your fault.   The answer are there you just need to find them.   Keep your priorities straight and keep your family close. You can't let everything else fall apart while you are dealing with a sick child. You still have other responsibilities. You have to be the glue that holds everything together.

Be grateful for the small successes and blessing that you are given. The healing may not happen in one day. Count the small successes and move on to find the big ones. Try to keep a positive attitude. Crying all day at your desk is not going to help anyone. And, it will likely get you fired. Limit the pity parties. Have one and then close it down. Lean on your support system instead of feeling sorry for yourself. Accept help from others when you need it. Talk to a friend when you need to and keep yourself strong and healthy so you can handle the stresses that lie ahead.

If you don't have a good support system – get one. Go to church or volunteer – you have to find a support system. You aren't going to be able to get through this alone.

My heart goes out to anyone who is effected or who has a love one who is effected by Crohn's Disease. It is a horrible disease that is hard to diagnose and is often misdiagnosed. There is no cure for Crohn's Disease – but there are effective treatments. You just have to keep searching until you find the one that is right for you.

Push forward for the answers and the help you need. And, do what you can to help others in need.

Thank you for reading my book. I hope you find these words to be a light in the dark tunnel of your journey through Crohn's Disease.

"Character cannot be developed in ease and quiet. Only through experience of trial and suffering can the soul be strengthened, ambition inspired, and success achieved,"

Helen Keller.

www.ingramcontent.com/pod-product-compliance
Lightning Source LLC
Chambersburg PA
CBHW031236250726
48655CB00005B/1979